MW01484811

KETO FAT BOMB

Delicious Fat Bombs In 10 Minutes Or Less

RYAN SMITH

ISBN: 9781095420164

TEXT COPYRIGHT © [RYAN SMITH]

TABLE OF CONTENT

INTRODUCTION

What Are Ketogenic Fat Bombs?

Many people are paranoid when it comes to eating fat. Although it has been public enemy number one for a long time, research has confirmed that fats can be extremely healthy. The only condition you need to fulfill is to choose the right type of fats. According to scientific reports, saturated fats, found in butter, coconut oil, cream cheese, and heavy cream influence our levels of good cholesterol. Proper levels good cholesterol improves our chances of avoiding and fighting heart disease, decreases our blood pressure, enhances our overall health, and, last but not least, gets our weight in order.

What a fat bomb contains.

1. Fat bombs are either sweet or savory. You'll find more recipes that swing towards the sweet side, but there are plenty savory recipe options available. A lot the sweeter recipes call for stevia, a low-calorie and no-carb sweetener. Many savory fat bombs are made with items like bacon, chicken, sausage, or salmon.

2. Fat bombs are small. These items are high in fat so, they are meant to be eaten in small servings. They will normally take the shape miniature muffins or a small ball.

3. Fat bombs can be made in large batches then stored in the refrigerator or freezer. Many fat bomb recipes make 10 or more servings at a time. They are ideal for people who want to cook once or twice a week and have healthy options on hand throughout the week. Fat bombs contain a high amount of fat and therefore will need to be kept cold when stored. These items are not meant to sit at room temperature for long periods. Fat bombs usually last for between 1 and 2 weeks when properly stored.

4. Fat bombs are high in healthy fats. These healthy fats are important when following a keto diet because they help lower levels inflammation in the body. Many keto fat bombs will have some form of coconut butter or coconut oil in them. These oils help solidify the fat bombs and make them less a mess to eat.

5. Fat bombs will often have seeds or nuts. Nuts are only meant to be eaten in small amounts due to the number carbohydrates they contain. This makes them ideal for fat bombs. Peanuts are not technically nuts, so the keto diet substitutes peanut butter with almond butter in their recipes.

Why Do You Need Ketogenic Fat Bombs?
As I mentioned, there are some fats that are bad, and these are called trans fats. On the other hand, there are 'good fats' that you should eat to help dissolve different vitamins, such as vitamins A, D, E, and K. Fat bombs also help reduce our bad cholesterol levels (LDL) and improve the amount good cholesterol (HDL).

Those you who are aiming to get rid extra pounds will surely be delighted to hear that fat bombs can help us get our weight under control. Each these recipes perfectly fits into ketogenic diet plans. Naturally, you will need to track your portion sizes; in other words, you can't eat too many these fat bombs.

Now that we are familiar with what fat bombs are let's move on to the recipes. I have included several recipes rich in healthy fats which also fit perfectly with a ketogenic diet.

Chapter 1: 14 Useful drinks you should know

1. Smoothie

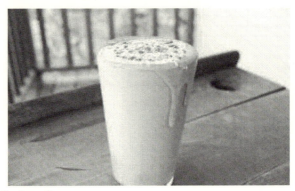

Serving: 1 fat bomb
Prep Time: 5 min

Ingredients

- 1/2 teaspoon and 1/8 teaspoon cinnamon, divided
- 6 drops liquid stevia
- 6 ice cubes
- 6 ounces half-and-half
- 1 tablespoon softened cream cheese
- 1 teaspoon vanilla extract

Instructions

- Add the half-and-half and cream cheese to a blender to combine.
- Add 1/2 teaspoon cinnamon, vanilla, and stevia then blend for 1 minute or until well mixed.
- Pour the ice cubes in and blend until the smoothie thickens.
- Sprinkle 1/8 teaspoon cinnamon on top and serve.

Nutrients per one serving: Calories: 283, Fat: 24g, Protein: 6g, Sodium: 116mg, Fiber: 1g, Carbohydrates: 9g, Sugar: 1g

2. Po Cha

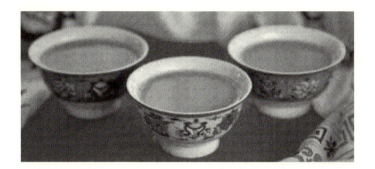

Serving: 2 people
Prep Time: 3 min
Cook Time: 8 min

Ingredients

- 2 tablespoons heavy cream
- 1/8 teaspoon sea salt
- 1 drop smoke flavor
- 4 cups water
- 2 tablespoons black tea leaves
- 2 tablespoons butter

Instructions

- Bring some water to a boil in a small saucepan then lower the heat to low.
- Add some tea leaves to the water and simmer for about 3 minutes, then strain.
- Combine the brewed tea with the remaining ingredients in a blender, then mix on high for about 3 minutes.
- Serve immediately.

Nutrients per one serving: Calories: 153, Fat: 17g, Protein: 0g, Sodium: 169mg, Fiber: 0g, Carbohydrates: 0g, Sugar: 0g

3. Creamy Coconut Smoothie

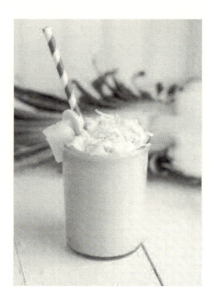

Serving: 1 fat bomb
Prep Time: 5 min

Ingredients

- 1⁄2 (13.5-ounce) can coconut milk
- 1 tablespoon unsweetened shredded coconut
- 6 drops liquid stevia
- 1 tablespoon powdered unflavored gelatin
- 1 tablespoon softened coconut oil
- 1 teaspoon vanilla extract
- 6 ice cubes

Instructions

- Pour the milk and gelatin into a blender then blend until combined.
- Add everything except for the ice cubes and blend for 1 minute or until well mixed.
- Pour the ice cubes in and blend until the smoothie thickens.
- Serve immediately.

Nutrients per one serving: Calories: 559, Fat: 57g, Protein: 10g, Sodium: 41mg, Fiber: 0g, Carbohydrates: 7g, Sugar: 1g

4. Creamy Mexican Hot Chocolate

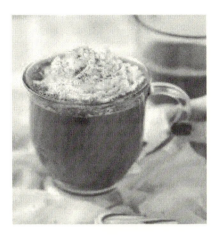

Serving: 2 people
Prep Time: 3 min
Cook Time: 5 min

Ingredients

- 1/8 teaspoon vanilla extract
- 1 cup water
- 1 cup heavy cream
- 2 teaspoons erythritol or granular Swerve, or 2 drops stevia glycerite
- 4 tablespoons unsweetened whipped cream
- 1/3 cup cocoa powder
- 1 teaspoon cinnamon

Instructions

- Combine all the ingredients except the whipped cream in a saucepan over very low heat.
- Stir frequently while heating until the cocoa powder is completely dissolved, about 5 minutes. Avoid boiling.
- When it's ready to serve, pour into 2 cups then top with whipped cream.

Nutrients per one serving: Calories: 538, Fat: 56g, Protein: 6g, Sodium: 63mg, Fiber: 5g, Carbohydrates: 17g, Sugar: 0g

5. Eggnog Smoothie

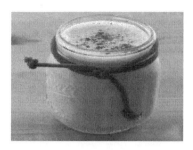

Serving: 2 fat bombs
Prep Time: 10 min

Ingredients

- 2 large eggs, the yolk and white separated
- 8 ounces heavy cream
- 8 drops liquid stevia
- 1 tablespoon granular Swerve
- 8 ice cubes
- 1/2 teaspoon vanilla extract
- 1 teaspoon nutmeg
- 1/8 teaspoon ground cloves
- 3/8 teaspoon cinnamon, divided

Instructions

- In a medium bowl, beat the egg whites using a hand mixer until stiff peaks form. Keep aside.
- In a separate large bowl, beat the yolks using a mixer until the color changes to pale yellow.
- Add vanilla, nutmeg, cream, cloves, 1/8 teaspoon cinnamon, stevia, and Swerve then stir well to combine.
- Fold the whites into the yolk mixture.
- Pour the mix into a blender with the ice cubes, then blend until the mixture thickens.
- Sprinkle 1/8 teaspoon cinnamon on the top every glass then serve immediately.

Nutrients per one serving: Calories: 468, Fat: 47g, Protein: 9g, Sodium: 113mg, Fiber: 1g, Carbohydrates: 5g, Sugar: 1g

6. Gingerbread Gem Smoothie

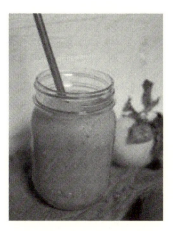

Serving: 1 fat bomb
Prep Time: 5 min

Ingredients
- 1/2 teaspoon ground ginger
- 1/2 teaspoon cinnamon
- 6 drops liquid stevia
- 6 ice cubes
- 6 ounces unsweetened almond milk
- 1 tablespoon powdered unflavored gelatin
- 1 tablespoon almond butter
- 1/2 teaspoon vanilla extract

Instructions
- Pour the milk and gelatin into a blender then blend until combined.
- Add everything except for the ice cubes and blend for 1 minute or until well mixed.
- Pour the ice cubes in and blend until the smoothie thickens.
- Serve immediately.

Nutrients per one serving: Calories: 221, Fat: 11g, Protein: 16g, Sodium: 174mg, Fiber: 3g, Carbohydrates: 16g, Sugar: 9g

7. Key Lime Pie Smoothie

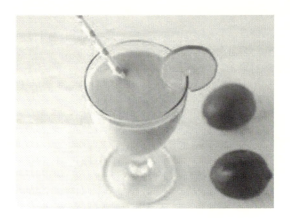

Serving: 1 fat bomb
Prep Time: 5 min

Ingredients

- 1 teaspoon lime zest
- 6 drops liquid stevia
- 6 ice cubes
- 6 ounces half-and-half
- 1 tablespoon powdered unflavored gelatin
- 1 teaspoon vanilla extract
- 2 tablespoons freshly squeezed key lime juice

Instructions

- Pour the half-and-half and gelatin into a blender then blend until combined.
- Add everything except for the ice cubes and blend for 1 minute or until well mixed.
- Pour the ice cubes in and blend until the smoothie thickens.
- Serve immediately.

Nutrients per one serving: Calories: 280, Fat: 20g, Protein: 12g, Sodium: 91mg, Fiber: 2g, Carbohydrates: 17g, Sugar: 3g

8. Matcha Madness Smoothie

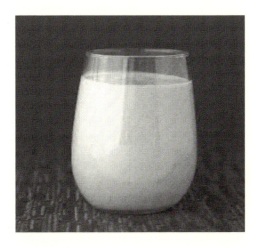

Serving: 1 fat bomb
Prep Time: 5 min

Ingredients
- 1/2 (13.5-ounce) can coconut milk
- 1 tablespoon matcha
- 6 drops liquid stevia
- Ice cubes
- 1 tablespoon powdered unflavored gelatin
- 2 tablespoons almond butter
- 1 teaspoon vanilla extract

Instructions
- Pour milk and gelatin into a blender then blend until combined.
- Add everything except for the ice cubes and blend for 1 minute or until well mixed.
- Pour the ice cubes in and blend until the smoothie thickens.
- Serve immediately.

Nutrients per one serving: Calories: 610, Fat: 57g, Protein: 19g, Sodium: 187mg, Fiber: 4g, Carbohydrates: 15g, Sugar: 4g

9. Peanut Butter Cup Smoothie

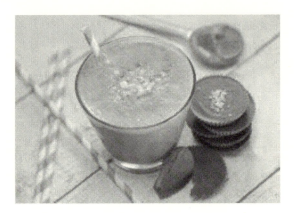

Serving: 1 fat bomb
Prep Time: 5 min

Ingredients

- 2 tablespoons cocoa powder
- 1 teaspoon vanilla extract
- 6 drops liquid stevia
- Ice cubes
- 1/2 (13.5-ounce) can coconut milk
- 1 tablespoon powdered unflavored gelatin
- 2 tablespoons peanut butter

Instructions

- Pour the milk and gelatin into a blender then blend until combined.
- Add everything except for the ice cubes and blend for 1 minute or until well mixed.
- Pour the ice cubes in and blend until the smoothie thickens.
- Serve immediately.

Nutrients per one serving: Calories: 622, Fat: 58g, Protein: 20g, Sodium: 189mg, Fiber: 6g, Carbohydrates: 18g, Sugar: 4g

10. Amaretto Chilled Coffee

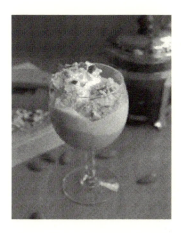

Serving: 2 fat bombs
Prep Time: 8 min

Ingredients
- 2 cups cooled brewed coffee
- 1/2 cup chilled heavy cream
- 1 teaspoon crumbled roasted almonds
- 4 teaspoons erythritol or granular Swerve /3 drops stevia glycerite, divided
- 4 drops divided amaretto flavor

Instructions
- Pour coffee into a medium bowl then add half the sweetener and half the amaretto flavor and mix.
- In a blender, add the chilled cream, the remaining amaretto flavor, and the remaining sweetener, then blend on high until the cream is whipped.
- Once it is ready to serve, pour the coffee mixture over the ice in 2 glasses.
- Spoon the whipped cream on top of the coffee mix. Decorate using chopped almonds.
- Serve immediately using a spoon and straw.

Nutrients per one serving: Calories: 421, Fat: 23g, Protein: 12g, Sodium: 55mg, Fiber: 0g, Carbohydrates: 45g, Sugar: 0g

11. Vanilla Smoothie

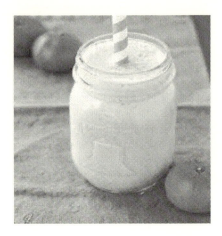

Serving: 1 fat bomb
Prep Time: 5 min

Ingredients

- The pulp of 1 vanilla bean, scraped
- 4 drops liquid stevia
- 6 ice cubes
- 6 ounces half-and-half
- 1 tablespoon powdered unflavored gelatin
- 1 teaspoon vanilla extract

Instructions

- Pour the half-and-half and gelatin into a blender then blend until combined.
- Add everything except for the ice cubes and blend for 1 minute or until well mixed.
- Pour the ice cubes in and blend until the smoothie thickens.
- Serve immediately.

Nutrients per one serving: Calories: 274, Fat: 19g, Protein: 11g, Sodium: 83mg, Fiber: 0g, Carbohydrates: 8g, Sugar: 1g

12. Vanilla Avocado Smoothie

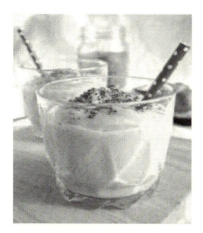

Serving: 1 fat bomb
Prep Time: 5 min

Ingredients

- 1/2 (13.5-ounce) can coconut milk
- 1 teaspoon vanilla extract
- 6 drops liquid stevia
- 4 ice cubes
- 1 tablespoon powdered unflavored gelatin
- 1 tablespoon ground flaxseed
- 1/2 pitted and peeled medium avocado

Instructions

- Pour gelatin, milk, and flaxseed into a blender then blend until combined.
- Add everything except for the ice cubes and blend for 1 minute or until well mixed.
- Pour the ice cubes in and blend until the smoothie thickens.
- Serve immediately.

Nutrients per one serving: Calories: 603, Fat: 57g, Protein: 14g, Sodium: 46mg, Fiber: 9g, Carbohydrates: 17g, Sugar: 1g

13. Vanilla Almond Butter Smoothie

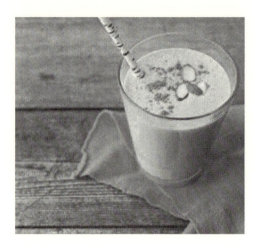

Serving: 1 fat bomb
Prep Time: 5 min

Ingredients

- 6 ounces unsweetened almond milk
- 1/4 teaspoon almond extract (optional)
- 6 drops liquid stevia
- 6 ice cubes
- 1 tablespoon powdered unflavored gelatin
- 2 tablespoons almond butter
- 1 teaspoon vanilla extract

Instructions

- Pour the milk and gelatin into a blender then blend until combined.
- Add everything except for the ice cubes and blend for 1 minute or until well mixed.
- Pour the ice cubes in and blend until the smoothie thickens.
- Serve immediately.

Nutrients per one serving: Calories: 316, Fat: 19g, Protein: 19g, Sodium: 248mg, Fiber: 3g, Carbohydrates: 17g, Sugar: 10g

14. Strawberry Vanilla Smoothie

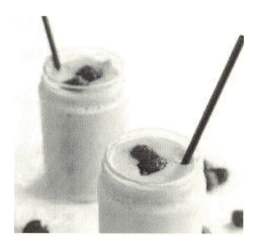

Serving: 1 fat bomb
Prep Time: 5 min

Ingredients

- 1⁄2 (13.5-ounce) can coconut milk
- 1⁄4 cup chopped fresh strawberries
- 6 drops liquid stevia
- 1 tablespoon powdered unflavored gelatin
- 1 tablespoon softened coconut oil
- 1 teaspoon vanilla extract
- 6 ice cubes

Instructions

- Pour the milk and gelatin into a blender then blend until combined.
- Add everything except for the ice cubes and blend for 1 minute or until well mixed.
- Pour the ice cubes in and blend until the smoothie thickens.
- Serve immediately.

Nutrients per one serving: Calories: 540, Fat: 54g, Protein: 10g, Sodium: 39mg, Fiber: 1g, Carbohydrates: 9g, Sugar: 2g

Chapter 2: How to have a delicious dish quickly and easily

15.Salted Caramel Almond

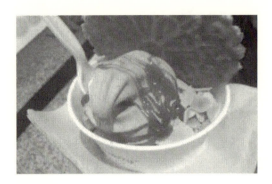

Serving: 12 fat bombs
Prep Time: 3 hours
Cook Time: 5 minutes

Ingredients
- 1/4 cup granular Swerve
- 2 teaspoons vanilla extract
- 12 whole almonds
- 1/4 cup butter
- 1 teaspoon coarse sea salt

Instructions
- Combine Swerve, butter, and vanilla in a small saucepan over medium heat. Stir frequently until the ingredients melt. Turn off heat.
- Place 1 almond in each mold of a 12-mold silicone candy tray.
- Add the mixture until the molds become about 3/4 full.
- Sprinkle salt on top of every fat bomb.
- Freeze until set, then serve from the freezer.

Nutrients per one serving: Calories: 64, Fat: 7g, Protein: 0g, Sodium: 296mg, Fiber: 0g, Carbohydrates: 1g, Sugar: 0g

16. Mocha Ice Bombs

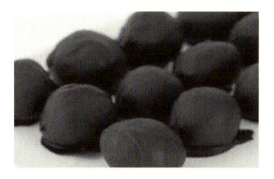

Serving: 12 people
Prep Time: 10 min

Ingredients
- 1/4cup powdered sweetener
- 2 tbsp. unsweetened cocoa
- 1/4cup strong coffee chilled
- 1cup cream cheese

Chocolate coating
- 70g melted chocolate
- 28g melted cocoa butter

Instructions
- Add coffee to the cream cheese, cocoa, and sweetener.
- Blend until smooth.
- To make an ice bomb shape, roll 2 tablespoons of the mocha ice bomb mixture to a ball, then place on a tray or plate lined with baking parchment.
- Chocolate coating
- Mix the melted chocolate and cocoa butter together.
- Roll every ice bomb in chocolate coating then place back on the lined tray/plate.
- Place in a freezer for about 2 hours.

Nutrients per one serving: Calories 127, Total fat 12.9g, Total Carbs 2.2g, Protein 1.9g

17. Low Carb Frozen Chocolate Chip Balls

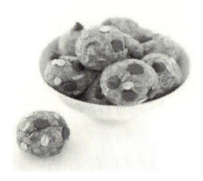

Serving: 16 people
Prep Time: 10 min

Ingredients

- 1/4 cup cocoa powder, unsweetened
- 1/2 cup Splenda (granulated)
- 1/2 cup low carb chocolate chips
- 1/4 cup water
- 1 Brick cream cheese
- 1 stick unsalted butter

Instructions

- Mix the cocoa powder and water until a thick paste is formed.
- Add the cream cheese, butter, cocoa mixture, and Splenda to a stand mixer then mix until smooth.
- Stir in chocolate chips.
- Form the mixture into 16 1" diameter balls. Put on a tray or pan lined with a silicone mat or baking parchment.
- Freeze for 1 hour then transfer to a lidded container.
- Remove from freezer about 10 minutes before eating.

Nutrients per one serving: Total carbs 5.7g, Fiber 06g, Protein 3.6g, Fat 34.6g, Magnesium 15mg, Potassium 94mg

18. Valentine's Day Keto Fat Bombs

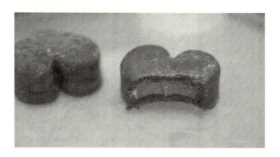

Serving: 4 people
Prep time: 2 min
Cook time: 2 min

Ingredients
- 1 teaspoon Cocoa Powder
- 2 Oz Dark Chocolate
- 8 Drops EZ-Sweetz
- 2 Oz. Almond Butter
- 2 Oz. Coconut Oil
- 1 Oz. Cream Cheese
- ½ Oz. Torani Sugar-Free Vanilla Syrup

Instructions
- Combine all items except the almond butter and microwave for about 30 seconds on high
- Stir the ingredients and microwave again. Repeat until the chocolate melts.
- Pour the base layer into the mold you are using
- Then use a spoon to dollop Almond Butter in the center of each mold.
- Fill the mold to the top with the chocolate mix
- Freeze until the chocolate becomes hard, then hard push these out of the mold
- Store in a fridge

Nutrients per one serving: Calories 297, Fat 30, Carbs 7, Fiber 3, Protein 5

19. Ice Cream

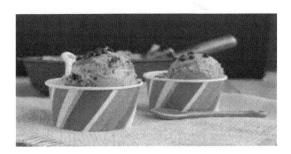

Serving: 5 people
Prep Time: 10 min

Ingredients
- 1/3 cup xylitol
- 1/3 cup flavor variation
- ¼ cup MCT oil
- 4 pastured eggs, whole
- 4 pastured eggs yolks
- 1/3 cup melted cacao butter
- 1/3 cup melted coconut oil
- 2 tsp vanilla bean powder
- 8-10 ice cubes

Instructions
- Add everything except the ice cubes to a high powered blender. Blend on high for about 2 minutes, or until creamy.
- As the blender runs, remove the top portion of the lid and drop in the ice cubes, one at a time, allowing the blender to run for about 10 seconds between every ice cube.
- Once you have added all the ice, pour the cold mixture into an ice cream maker and churn it on high for about 20-30 minutes, as per the ice cream maker directions.
- Serve this immediately as a soft-serve or scoop it into 9 * 5 loaf pan and freeze for about 45 minutes. Store while covered in freezer for about a week.

Nutrients per one serving: Calories: 431, Calories from Fat: 399, Saturated Fat: 34 g, Total Fat: 44.3, Sodium: 56 mg, Carbs: 3.4 g, Cholesterol: 299> mg, Dietary Fiber: 1.6 g, Protein: 7.7 g, Net Carbs: 1.8 g

20.Blueberry Cheesecake Popsicles

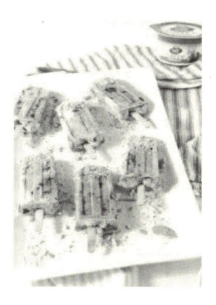

Serving: 10 people
Prep Time: 5 minutes

Ingredients

- 8 Tbsps. light cream cheese
- 6 Tbsps. icing sugar
- 2 cups fresh blueberries
- 30 Tbsps. Cool Whip

Instructions

- Puree the blueberries, cream cheese, and icing sugar in a blender until smooth.
- Gently fold in the whipped topping.
- Spoon into popsicle molds then freeze until firm.
- Run the mold under hot water to loosen the popsicles so they are easy to release.

Nutrients per one serving: 83 calories, 3 fat, 1 protein, 15 carbs.

21. Blueberry Fat Bombs

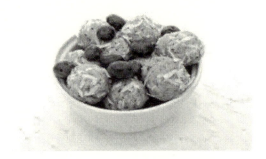

Serving: 24 fat bombs
Prep Time: 10 min

Ingredients
- 1 stick butter (4 oz.)
- Scant cup blueberries
- 3/4 c. coconut oil
- 4 oz. softened cream cheese
- ¼ c. coconut cream
- Sweetener to taste

Instructions
- In a food processor, place the coconut cream, berries, and soft cream cheese.
- Puree until smooth.
- In a saucepan over low heat, melt the coconut oil and butter.
- Let cool for about 5 minutes, then add to the food processor and puree again until smooth.
- Slowly, add the sweetener of your choice while tasting and adjusting to your liking.
- Transfer the mixture into molds leaving space at the top.
- Freeze for one hour and enjoy.
- You can also freeze them in suitable plastic bags.

Nutrients per one serving: 116 calories, 44g protein, 13g fat, 1.02g carbs 84g NET CARBS, .18g fiber

22. Cream Cheese Fat Bombs

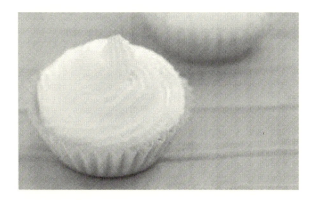

Serving: 2 balls
Prep Time: 10 minutes
Cook Time: 5 minutes

Ingredients
- Sugar-free Jell-O, 1 package, or pudding mix
- 1 8oz package Kraft Philadelphia cream cheese

Instructions
- Cut the cream cheese into 16 squares.
- Put the Jell-O or pudding mix into a small bowl.
- Cover each cream cheese square on all the sides using the mix.
- Roll into a ball.
- Keep covered with a plastic wrap inside your fridge.

Nutrients per one serving: 105 calories, 9 g fat, 1 carb, and 3 g protein

23. Chocolate Macadamia Fat Bomb

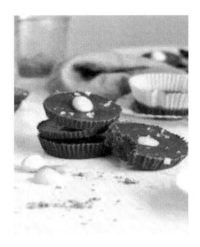

Serving: 6 people
Prep Time: 5 minutes
Cook Time: 5 minutes

Ingredients

- 4 oz. Chopped macadamias
- ¼ cup Heavy cream or coconut oil
- 2 oz. Cocoa Butter
- 2 Tbs unsweetened cocoa powder
- 2 Tbs Swerve

Instructions

- Melt the cocoa butter in a small saucepan.
- Add cocoa powder and Swerve then mix well.
- Add the macadamias then stir in well.
- Add cream, then mix well, bring it back to temperature.
- Pour in molds or paper candy cups.
- Allow to cool, then place in a fridge to harden.
- Store at room temperature.

Nutrients per one serving: Calories 267, Fat 28gm, Net carbs 3gm, Protein 3gm

24.Happy Almond Bombs

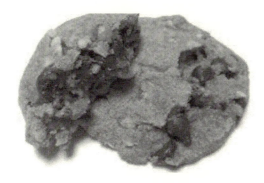

Serving: 4 people
Prep Time: 5 minutes
Cook Time: 5 minutes

Ingredients
- 4 tablespoons almond butter
- 1oz cream cheese
- 4 tablespoons coconut butter
- 1 tablespoon cocoa powder
- 2 tablespoons sugar-free syrup
- 16g dark chocolate

Instructions
- Add everything except the coconut butter in a microwave-safe dish.
- Microwave in 15 seconds intervals, stirring every time, until the chocolate and cream cheese have melted and all ingredients have fully incorporated.
- Add coconut butter and mix.
- Spoon the batter into 12 portions in a mini-muffin tray.
- Pop these into a freezer for about 1 hour to set. Enjoy.

Nutrients per one serving: Calories 86, Total fat 7g, Total carbs 3g, protein 2g, cholesterol 3mg, sodium 21mg

25. Blackberry Coconut Fat Bombs

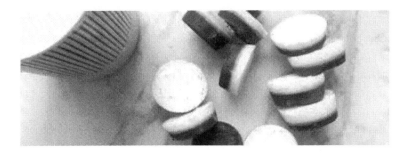

Serving: 6 people
Total Time: 10 minutes

Ingredients

- 1 cup coconut butter
- 1/2 cup frozen blackberries can
- 1/2 teaspoon Sweat leaf Stevia drops
- 1/4 teaspoon vanilla powder or a 1/2 teaspoon vanilla extract
- 1 tablespoon lemon juice
- 1 cup coconut oil

Instructions

- Place the coconut oil, coconut butter, and blackberries in a pot then heat over medium heat until well combined.
- In a food processor or small blender, add the berry mix and the remaining ingredients. Mix until smooth.
- Spread out on a small pan lined with a parchment paper
- Refrigerate for one hour.
- Remove from the container then cut into squares.
- Store while covered in a refrigerator.

Nutrients per one serving: Calories 170 Calories from Fat 168, Total Fat 18.7g, Total carbohydrates 3g, Dietary Fiber 2.3g, Protein 1.1g

26. Ginger Fat Bombs

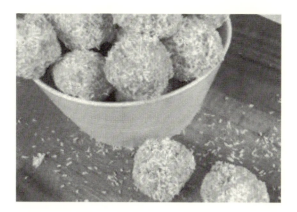

Serving: 10 people
Prep Time: 10 min

Ingredients

- 75g / 2.6oz coconut butter
- 75g / 2.6oz coconut oil
- 25g / 1oz shredded/desiccated coconut
- 1 tsp granulated sweetener
- 1/2-1 tsp ginger powder

Instructions

- Mix all the ingredients in a pouring jug until the sweetener dissolves.
- Pour into silicon molds or ice block trays then refrigerate for around 10 minutes.

Nutrients per one serving: Calories 120, Total Fat 12.8g, Fiber 1.4g, Sugars 0.1g, Protein 0.5g

27. Lemon Clouds

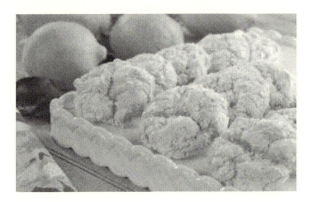

Serving: 16 bombs
Prep Time: 10 min

Ingredients
- 1 lemon, squeezed
- 1 tsp lemon extract
- Sweetener to taste
- Silicone mold or ice cube tray
- 4 tbsps. butter
- 4 tbsps. virgin coconut oil
- 2oz cream cheese
- 4 tbsps. heavy cream

Instructions
- Begin with the cream cheese, heating it in short bursts.
- Add the butter and coconut oil, then whisk until well blended.
- Add the cream last then whisk.
- Squeeze in the lemon, watching for the pesky seeds. Add extract if needed.
- Sweeten to taste.
- Carefully pour into the tray then balance in the freezer overnight.
- Pop them from the tray in the next morning.

Nutrients per one serving: Calories: 74.7, Fat: 8g, Protein: 0.3g, Carbs: 0.7g, Fiber: 0.8g, Sugars: 0.3g

28. Orange Pecan Butter Fat Bombs

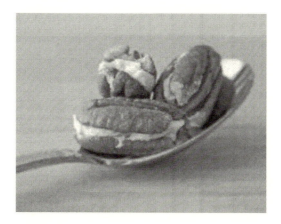

Serving: 2 people
Prep Time: 10 min

Ingredients
- 4 pecan halves
- 1/2 tbsp. unsalted grass-fed butter
- 1/2 tsp orange zest, finely grated
- 1 pinch sea salt

Instructions
- Toast the pecans at 350° in an oven for 8-10 minutes, then keep aside to cool.
- Soften butter, then add orange zest and mix well until smooth and creamy.
- Spread half the butter-orange mixture in two pecan halves. Sprinkle using sea salt then enjoy.

Nutrients per one serving: Calories 89, Net carbs 1

29. Cheesy Pesto Fat Bombs

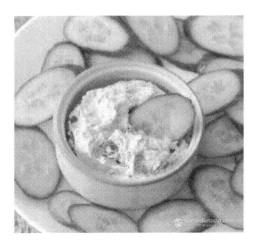

Serving: 8 people
Prep Time: 5 min

Ingredients

- 10 sliced olives
- Salt, pepper to taste (optional)
- 1 cup full-fat cream cheese
- 2 tbsps. basil pesto
- ½ cup grated Parmesan cheese

Instructions

- Place all ingredients in a bowl using a spatula until well combined.
- Slice a cucumber or the other fresh vegetable which you are planning to serve it with.
- Place remaining dip in an airtight container in a fridge for a week.

Nutrients per one serving: Total Carbs 1.6g, Fiber 0.3g, Protein 4.3g, Fat 12.9g, Magnesium 37mg, Potassium 50mg

30. Cream Cheese and Peanut Butter Fat Bomb

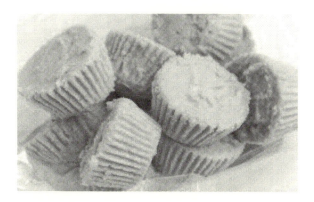

Serving: 14 pieces
Prep Time: 10 min

Ingredients

- 2 Tablespoons sour cream
- 4 Tablespoons softened cream cheese
- 1 cup heavy whipping cream
- 3 Tablespoons BP2 peanut butter, powdered
- 2 Tablespoons Splenda

Instructions

- Whip heavy whipping cream until it is light and airy.
- Add the remaining ingredients and mix well.
- Spoon into a silicone candy mold tray to make 14 portions, then freeze overnight.
- Serve them partially frozen or allow them to defrost completely for a fluffy treat.

Nutrients per one serving: Calories 82, Total fat 8g, Cholesterol 24mg, Sodium 29mg, Totals carbs 1g, Protein 1g

31. Chocolate Mousse

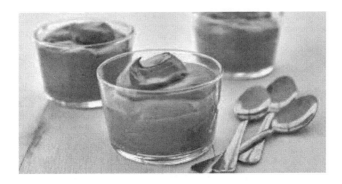

Serving: 4 people
Prep Time: 5 min

Ingredients
- ½ tsp cinnamon
- 6-12 drops liquid stevia extract
- Shredded coconut for garnish
- 1 cup creamed coconut milk
- 3 tbsps. raw cocoa powder

Instructions
- Put the can of coconut milk in the fridge overnight. Once thick, pour into a bowl.
- Whip in raw cocoa powder.
- Add in cinnamon and stevia.
- Whip until smooth and creamy.
- Place in serving glasses, then garnish using a pinch of shredded coconut. Enjoy!

Nutrients per one serving: Total Carbs 13.5g, Fiber 5.8g, Protein 6.2g, Fat 42.9g, Magnesium 75mg, Potassium 520mg

32. Chocolate Fat Bombs

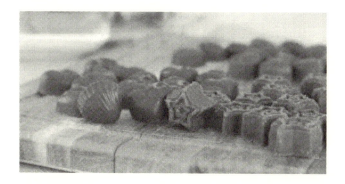

Serving: 14 people
Prep Time: 10 min

Ingredients

- 125g / 4.5oz coconut oil
- 25g / 1oz unsweetened cocoa powder
- 1 tbsp. granulated sweetener
- 1-2 tbsps. tahini paste
- 25g / 1oz walnut halves

Instructions

- Warm the coconut oil until it melts.
- Add everything except the walnuts and allow to cool so the ingredients do not settle and sink to the bottom your fat bomb.
- Pour into ice cube trays then refrigerate until it is semi-set.
- Once it's almost set, put half a walnut on top of every fat bomb.

Nutrients per one serving: Calories 119, Total fat 12.6g, Total Carbs 1.2g, Protein 1.4g

33. Peanut Butter Fudge

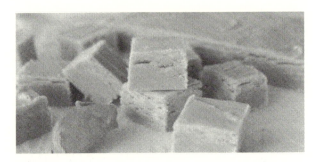

Serving: 12 people
Prep Time: 5 min

Ingredients

- 1 cup unsweetened peanut butter
- 1/4 cup unsweetened cocoa powder
- 1 cup coconut oil
- 1/4 cup vanilla almond milk, unsweetened
- Pinch salt (optional)
- 2 teaspoons vanilla liquid stevia (optional)
- 2 tablespoons coconut oil, melted
- 2 tablespoons Swerve

Instructions

- Slightly melt/soften the peanut butter and coconut oil in the microwave or over low heat on a stove.
- Add the mix and remaining ingredients to a blender.
- Blend until well combined.
- Pour into a loaf pan with lined with parchment paper.
- Refrigerate for 2 hours until set.
- If you are using chocolate sauce, whisk the ingredients together then drizzle over the fudge after it has set.

Nutrients per one serving: Calories 287, Fat 29.7g, Carbs 4g, Sugar 0.7g, Sodium 4mg, Fiber 1.4g, Protein 5.4g

34. Buttered Bacon Fat Bomb

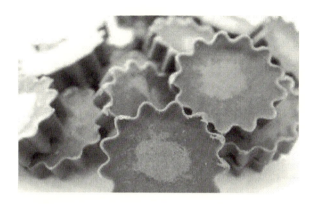

Serving: 3 fat bombs
Prep Time: 2 min

Ingredients

- 1 bacon slice
- 2 toasted & chopped pecan halves
- 1/16 serving Keto Craisin
- 1 tablespoon unsalted Kerrygold butter
- 1 pinch granulated garlic (optional)

Instructions

- Divide your bacon into 3 parts. Slather each using 1 teaspoon of Kerrygold unsalted butter.
- Press the butter side into your pecan pieces.
- Top each using Keto Craisin.

Nutrients per one serving: 158 Calories, 2g Protein, 17g Fat, 1g Carbohydrate, 1g Effective Carbs, trace Dietary Fiber

35. Mocha Vanilla Fat Bomb Pops

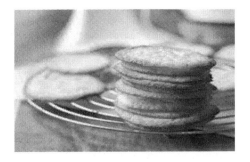

Serving: 6 people
Prep Time: 10 min

Ingredients

- 2 tbsps. heavy cream
- 1/2 tsp vanilla extract
- 4 tbsps. coconut oil
- 1/2 tbsp. unsweetened cocoa powder
- 4 tbsps. unsalted butter
- 1/2 tsp coffee extract
- Stevia, to taste

Instructions
Make vanilla layer:

- Soften butter in a microwave until liquefied.
- Add the heavy cream and stir. Keep aside.
- Once cooled, add vanilla, then blend well.
- Pour vanilla mixture into muffin liners/tins. Place into refrigerator until firm.

Make mocha layer:

- Mix coconut oil, coffee extract, cocoa powder, and stevia.
- Remove the vanilla layer from the fridge, then pour in mocha mixture, filling the cups to the top.
- Add popsicle sticks then freeze for 20 to 30 minutes.

Nutrition information per serving: 167 Calories; trace Protein, 19g Fat, .5g Dietary Fiber, 1g Carbohydrate

Chapter 3: A thing you need to know before you make keto fat bombs

You need to know which food or drink to use at the right time. We classify these recipes into 4 groups to help you use them better.

Group 1: Breakfast
-Smoothie
-Po Cha
-Creamy Coconut Smoothie
-Creamy Mexican Hot Smoothie
-Eggnog Smoothie
-Gingerbread Gem Smoothie
-Key Lime Pie Smoothie
-Matcha Madness Smoothie
-Peanut Butter Cup Smoothie
-Amaretto Chilled Coffee
-Vanilla Avocado Smoothie
-Vanilla Almond Butter Smoothie
-Strawberry Vanilla Smoothie

Group 2: Lunch
-Salted Caramel Almond
-Mocha Ice Bombs
-Low-carb Frozen Chocolate Chip Balls

Group 3: Dinner
-Valetine's Day Keto Fat Bombs
-Ice Cream
-Blueberry Cheesecake Popsicles
-Blueberry Fat Bombs
-Cream Cheese Fat Bombs
-Chocolate Macadamia Fat Bombs

-Happy Almond Bombs
-Blackberry Coconut Fat Bomb

Group 4: Dessert

-Ginger Fat Bombs
-Lemon Clouds
-Orange Pecan Butter Fat Bombs
-Chessy Pesto Fat Bombs
-Cream Cheese and Peanut Butter Fat Bombs
-Chocolate Mousse
-Chocolate Fat Bombs
-Peanut Butter Fudge
-Buttered Bacon Fat Bomb
-Mocha Vanilla Fat Bomb Pops

CHECK OUT OTHER BOOKS

Go here to check out other related books that might interest you:

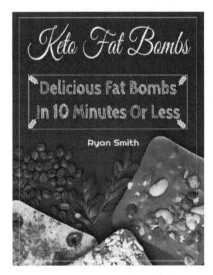

KETO FAT BOMB
Delicious Fat Bombs In 10 Minutes Or Less
https://www.amazon.com/dp/B07NK8NRRN

Made in the USA
Middletown, DE
06 April 2023

28382646R00026